CONTENTS

DON'T TAKE THIS PANDEMIC SITTING DOWN

By

Daniel Sheridan

* Cover Illustration by Daniel Sheridan

INTRODUCTION

An introduction seems necessary because there is always the possibility that someone will read this book and find fault with the whole idea of what might, to them, seem to be a lazy way to maintain a measure of health through the pandemic.

My whole reason for writing this book is not to encourage laziness but to acknowledge that some are unable to do more. This could be due to their current state of health or due to depression from the constant flow of bad news lately. Some people just need our empathy.

I have extreme respect for doctors and everyone in the health field and am aware that they may feel that this book may encourage laziness which would seem to be a bad approach to good health. However, not everyone is at the same stage of mobility or even general physical wellness. My reason for writing this book is to encourage anyone, at any stage to just do something. I am merely offering a simple alternative; a beginning from which anyone can progress to any measure of fitness one wishes.

DON'T JUST SIT STILL FOR THE PANDEMIC

Chapter 1

You can rightly ask, "Who am I to write such a book on this subject?" My answer would be, "Nobody special, just the average guy."

And THAT is what makes me just the right guy to write this book. I'm about 6 feet tall. Married. I did weigh about 205 till I cut down on bread and sugar, and like everyone else have had my life impacted by the recent pandemic.

I do enjoy reading though and have come across a variety of ideas that I thought might help me, as well as others gain a measure of physical wellness while being stuck at home in these most unusual circumstances.

Whether working or not, our time at home has increased. Most of our social contact has now been limited to screen-time, and consequently our lives have become increasingly sedentary. This could be dangerous on several levels. Not only are we likely to gain weight from less walking, but we tend to feel a need to entertain ourselves more by means of tv, movies or games. For some, after months of this routine, it has even led to depression.

I don't claim to have all the answers, but It seems obvious that we need to fight the tendency toward inertia. We **can't** be a couch potato and come out at the end of this pandemic as healthy as we were going into it.

So, for any that don't have a plan at all, here is one from just your average guy who cares enough about himself, his family and you to come up with some kind of plan. In fact, my purpose is to come up with a minimal plan, one that can be followed by **anybody,** regardless of their present state of health. I am taking the time and effort to put it to paper for the good of all that wish to read it, in the hopes that it might help some.

CHAPTER 2

ALL THE SAME

Despite our obvious differences in height, weight, color or gender we are all basically the same and that is the reason that I have written this book with a minimal amount of effort in mind. This way, the exercises can be practiced by anyone, except those with serious mobility issues.

So, let's start it all off with one of the most basic things that we all do. **We all breathe.** But, perhaps we can learn to breath better.

The first thing to learn is to breath in through your nose. In general, it would be best to make this your regular practice since this is where your built-in air filters are.

Occasionally, maybe several times during the day, take the time to be aware of your breathing and breathe deeply, letting your belly rise. Hold the breath for a few seconds then expel it slowly through the mouth. Try this for between three to five times till you are able to do more repetitions. This will help you relax. The body needs tension-free time to heal, especially when almost all the news in the media is negative.

You don't have to be aware of every breath you take but just attempting to fit this into your schedule two to four times a day may help you relieve quite a bit of tension.

CHAPTER 3

MIND THE BODY

Cut the Sugar and Bread

Take the time to look after the body you were given. Don't worry, I'm not going to make this difficult. Like I said at the start, my goal is to keep the program to the absolute minimum so that anyone, myself included, will maintain a degree of health without being discouraged by too much effort, at least, in the beginning. If you wish to intensify the program, more power to you. Please feel free to do more breathing or physical exercises as you wish and, of course, with your doctors permission.

At the start I told you that I lost quite a few pounds just by slowing my intake of sugar and bread. I know that I could have accomplished so much more by dropping sugar and bread entirely, but I just don't have that kind of will power at the moment. I had occasionally done a few push-ups or crunches but would just seem to forget to do it after a few days which meant that the benefit came and went. So, just for the sake of testing this method I will not do any exercising other than mentioned in this book, after which we can compare my before and after weights.

As I said my weight had gone up to about 205 pounds. There was no real change in weight till noticing what was happening as my hand went to my mouth. That was about a month and half ago. Just by being more mindful of the amount of sugar and bread I was consuming my weight has dropped to 194 pounds as of today, July 26, 2020. So why do I need more when this alone seems to be working? The answer is that I am still not comfortable. I still have a "dad belly" that hangs a bit over the belt, and I can't bend over like I used to. Does this all sound familiar? I am aware that I felt best at 180 to 185 pounds so that is my goal.

Sometimes it's just a matter of making better choices. When I want to sit and unconsciously dip an endless amount of cookies in coffee, (just one of my bad habits), I now have been able to take a second to make a choice. A few pretzel sticks or 1 bag of popcorn may not be the most healthy choice but it's better than basically pouring sugar down your throat. If you just have to go for the cookies only bring a maximum of five to the chair with you that way if you choose to eat more, you at least have to get out of your chair.

Sugar and bread are just some of the things that seem to make our lives more pleasant so giving them up isn't easy. I haven't accomplished it yet, though I'm well aware of my need to. Considering how much even slowing my intake of them has helped me I would absolutely recommend it to you. By the way, I have noticed an improvement in my mental clarity and memory function since diminishing just these two ingredients. I hope to eventually cut them out of my life entirely, except for an occasional piece of cheesecake, maybe. I have made it a goal to continue down this road and hope you will too.

There is one thing I would like to add here related to eating. Stop eating when your full. The temptation to eat more will leave in about 10 minutes and if you can resist till then your stomach will thank you. It's probably one of the quickest ways to succeed at weight-loss. Admittedly, I'm not really good at this one, but I'm working on it.

CHAPTER 4

VERY EASY EXERCISES

Yay! Easy is good. Right? For someone that can't get out of the house much and doesn't want to get fat it sure is. But again, the goal is not just to survive the pandemic without getting depressed and heavier, but to come out on the other side of it happier, healthier and skinnier.

The body was made to move. Although covid-19 makes it more difficult, we must take time to exercise even if only during commercials, in the beginning, if we really want some improvement in our life after the pandemic is over.

You don't have to give up T.V. or Facebook. Just remember to take a commercial break and get up and out of the chair. While you're out of the chair **move!** Staying still is your enemy! Try these simple things. I'm in my 60's so these steps are **easy!**

As a reminder, these exercises are simple and quick enough to be done during a 5 minute break or less. Do them when taking some time during television commercials, or between Facebook pages. If you wish, do them throughout the day for even more benefit. Just **do them!** You will benefit only as much as you want to. Even if you are older, unmotivated, or just plain can't move easily try these simple exercises before the metaphorical rust sets in and you can't.

STRETCH while standing

Just Place your feet and bend to your left. Come back to center. Bend to your right. Return to center.

Start doing this just once or twice during every other commercial break. The objective is to get out of the chair and let the blood flow.

Try to alternate the side stretch with a front to back stretch. Don't go bend to far back and support your back with your hands on your sides, fingers turned toward the kidneys and thumbs aimed forward on your side.

After a week or so you can try a complete rotation from the waist while bending forward.

While standing you might also try bending down as far as you can then standing straight. If you can, stand beside your easy chair. Place your hand on the side of the chair and stand up on the balls of your feet stretching your calves. Hold this position for a few seconds and repeat a couple of times.

STRETCH while sitting

Stretching doesn't always have to be done standing up. While watching your favorite show bend your head slowly to the left and then to the right. Do the same thing forward and back. Then, rotate from the neck clockwise and counterclockwise.

While sitting, bend from the waist. Stretch to the left, then to the right. Stretch your arms above your head as far as you can. Don't forget to bring them back down or you won't be able to eat that donut. (just kidding!)

Try lifting your left leg and stretch your feet forward and back then return your leg. Now try the same with your right leg. Repeat this a couple times and you might even feel like turning the T.V. off and doing something else.

WALK

Don't worry. I don't mean around the block. I'm just talking about doing it in place. How many commercials do you get in a typical television show? If you just walked in place during every commercial break you may find you've walked a mile by the end of the day. If that's too boring for you how about walking around your chair or around the room. Maybe even, after you do this for a while you might be able to jog in place, or later, even run in place. The more you do, the more you'll lose. But you will also gain by releasing endorphins and those make you feel happy!

By the way, if in time you do get to feeling well enough to walk around your yard or the block, do it! As you lose each pound you will enjoy life just a little more.

TWIST

This one is only to be done if your physically capable.

Stand up, put your hands on your waist or, if you need stability, on the side of your chair and **do the twist.** Do it at one level loosely bending your knees and lifting the heels, or if your not self-conscious and just want to have more fun while doing it and benefit even more, do the dance. Twist left and right while bending the knees and going higher and lower. **Dance!** Twist and Shout!

ARM WRESTLE YOURSELF

I remember as a child looking at my comic books and finding the Charles Atlas ads and not wanting to be that 90 lb. weakling. I never had the money to buy the course but have since learned of some of his techniques. John McSweeney's Tiger Moves are similar and very beneficial.

Borrowing just the simplest ideas from these masters and others that I've read I would like to give you, the reader, something that will improve muscle tone quickly. You will be amazed at how quickly improvement will be made with so little work and time. All of these will be exercises you can practice from your chair while watching your favorite program. If your improvement becomes as great as I'm sure it will you may wish, at that time, to invest some time and money in one of the aforementioned books or programs.

   1. Sit up straight and hold your left arm out while bending at the elbow. Lift your right arm and bend it, grabbing your left hand. Now push your left hand as though you are performing an arm wrestle with your right hand, while your right hand resists it. Don't push too much, especially in the beginning. Do this for about 3 seconds at first.

Now switch to the right arm. Lift it as though doing an arm wrestle in the air. Hold and resist with your left hand and arm.

Repeat this about three times at first

2. Sit up straight and hold your hands together. (Love yourself!). Lift your hands in front of your body and press. You should feel your chest tightening.

Hold this for about three seconds and release. Try to repeat this 3 times. Again, if you wish repeat a few more times later. The goal is to do more than you were while not becoming so sore that you don't want to do it anymore.

CRUNCH

I'm not referring to conventional crunches. You don't even have to leave your chair for this one.

While sitting turn your hands palm up and close them into fists. Lift them up to about shoulder height. Now with some pressure pull your elbows down to your sides as if you just won something awesome and your saying, "YES!" While your doing that, contract your abdominal muscles and lean forward just a little bit. Three times should be enough for now. But gradually increasing the repetitions to 10 would be a great goal.

As you can see, none of these exercises are difficult, but doing them faithfully can make a big difference in your life, especially now when it would be so easy to do nothing. Your future self would be so happy to thank you today if it were possible.

CHAPTER 5

A Few Extras That Will Help

1. **Get plenty of sleep**. This one is difficult for me, but I'm well aware of its importance and so would be negligent if I didn't encourage you to accomplish it. Seven to Eight hours are best but aim for at least six. Your body needs time to heal from life's onslaughts whether physical or mental.

2. **Get your vitamins**. Do some research and choose carefully. Check with your doctor and don't overdo it. Personally, I feel that vitamin D and vitamin C are very important. I know that they will not prevent me from getting the coronavirus, but it is my belief that they help keep me healthier till and if it happens.

3. **Change position while sitting**. It's too easy to become so absorbed in a movie or book that we forget to move. This is bad for your circulation and may result in pain that would keep you from wanting to do anything later. Just be aware of yourself and your position in space. Do you need to sit back a little further in your chair? Try crossing your legs or if you are already then cross them the other way. Lean a little to the left and then after a while lean a little to the right. Are you sitting straight back? Try to lean forward for a minute or two and then sit back. The whole idea is to keep the blood and lymph moving.

4. **Take your wallet out of your back pocket.** I'm guilty of this,

and then wonder why my leg's feel restless. I'm not saying this is a cause of restless leg syndrome, but when I think to remove my wallet from my back pocket, I do find that I'm bothered by it much less.

5. **Massage your hands and feet.** Take your shoes off. Rub your feet, ankles and legs. Don't forget to rub your hands, wrists and arms. This is an investment in your health. Whether you call it shiatsu or reflexology it will at the very least relax tension.

6. A Few Other Things

I didn't mention it till now because it's become so much of a political issue but wear your mask anytime your around other people. This pandemic won't go on forever so forget your pride and wear it for your sake and the sake of those you love.

Here's a hodgepodge of other things that I've added as a reminder to myself and anyone else that may care to have a to do list to make things a little easier.

- Rotate your shoulders forward, then backward.
- Rotate your head in a circular motion first one direction, then the other.
- Rotate your wrists.
- Rotate your feet.
- Stretch your fingers.
- Reach for your toes while sitting.
- During commercials mute the sound, close your eyes and listen to your breathing.
- Drink water not soda.
- Eat some fruit.
- This one may seem silly, but there are those that get so

involved in games, movies or books that taking the time to get up to go to the bathroom is the last thing on their mind. Take the time to stop, get up and go to the bathroom. Your kidneys will thank you.

CONCLUSION

Incidentally it is now, (August/8/2020), a little over a week, since starting this book and my weight is now close to 190 lbs. I have done nothing other than what is outlined in this book and am confident that I will reach my goal soon. If I can do it so can you!

There is no reason that we can't come out of any bad situation better or healthier than we were going into it. We must persevere though. Be willing to put forth some effort. This book is outlining a start, but don't let that be the end of it. If you get feeling better as a result of this writing, as I believe you will, then don't stop! Keep progressing. Let this be a new beginning for you.